TABLE OF CONTENTS

1 INTRODUCTION

If you have sudden painful, swollen joints in your toes or feet or perhaps your ankles, knees, fingers, hands, or elbows, you may be experiencing gout. Gout is a condition caused by a buildup of uric acid causing inflammation and irritation in your joints resulting in pain, swelling, and other symptoms. If you are dealing with gout, know that this is not a life sentence. There are some simple natural support strategies that you can try to improve your health.

2   OVERVIEW OF GOUT

Gout is a type of arthritis. It is a condition caused by accumulation and buildup of uric acid from poor dietary habits and metabolic issues. Gout causes damage and swelling in various joints of the body. When uric acid builds up in your body, it forms crystals called urates. Urates are rather sharp and can penetrate into your joints causing irritation and inflammation.

Gout usually affects your feet, particularly, your big toe. It can also affect your ankles, wrists, knees, elbows, and fingers. It is characterized by pain and swelling. You may experience gout attacks that are sudden and intense as if your foot is on fire.

Some people with gout may experience asymptomatic gout without symptoms. In most cases of acute gout, you can expect the following symptoms from the quick buildup of uric acid):

- Intense joint pain
- Swelling
- Lingering discomfort
- Inflammation
- Redness
- Heat
- Stiffness
- Limited range of motion

You may notice these symptoms in your toes (especially your big toe), feet, knees, wrist, elbows, and fingers. Acute gout symptoms may last for 3 to

10 days. You won't be experiencing symptoms of gout until your next gout attack.

Untreated gout may turn chronic, however, cause hard lumps called tophi to develop in your joints, skin, and surrounding tissue. Since tophi can cause permanent joint damage, addressing acute gout, and reducing your risks of gout attacks is critical.

2.2   MAJOR CAUSES FOR GOUT

Gout affects over 3 million people in the United States. Men, women after menopause, those with kidney disease, those with hypertension, hyperlipidemia, and diabetes are more likely to be affected. Gout may develop for a variety of reasons, including one or more of these major causes of gout:

Genetic Tendency

Your genetics may increase your chances of developing gout. Gout tends to run in families. If you have one or more people in your family with gout, your risk of developing gout yourself is higher.

While you cannot change your family history, gout may develop for more than one reason. If you have a family history of gout, it is particularly important that you pay attention to other major causes of gout that you can control easier through a healthy diet and lifestyle.

Poor Blood Sugar and Insulin Resistance

Insulin resistance happens when your cells in your fat, liver, and muscles are unable to respond to insulin properly and cannot handle all the glucose from your blood. This forces your pancreas to make more and more insulin to help glucose to enter your cells. Insulin resistance and poor blood sugar can increase your risk of diabetes which can increase your risk of gout.

According to a 1998 study published in the Annals of Epidemiology and a 2013 study published in PLoS, those with gout also have an increased risk of insulin resistance and diabetes. Insulin resistance may also increase inflammation in your body which further aggravates your gout symptoms.

Poor Purine Metabolism

Uric acid forms from two major biochemical patterns. The most commonly associated pathway that doctors discuss when it comes to gout is through purine metabolism. Purines are molecules that are formed by a grouping of nucleic acids.

Pure purine metabolism and foods high in purine, such as shellfish, fish, red meat, turkey, organ meats, gravies, and soups may increase your risk of gout. Purine converts into uric acid in your body. The problem is that if your kidneys are unable to flush the excess uric acid, it can create a buildup in your bloodstream and end up depositing in your joints leading to gout.

Gout is the most common condition seen in those with poor purine metabolism. According to a 1998 study in Biochemistry Journal, purine metabolism abnormalities can increase the risk of both gout and neurological dysfunction.

In general, some people don't tolerate these foods as well as others

Poor Fructose Metabolism

Poor fructose metabolism and eating or drinking foods or drinks high in fructose, especially high-fructose corn syrup may also cause gout. This second biochemical pathway indicated that fructose triggers the body's production of uric acid from and important energy molecule adenosine triphosphate.

According to a 2010 study published in the Journal of American Medical Association, participants who drank one fructose-rich beverage a day were 74 percent more likely to develop gout than those who only had one high-fructose drink a month. Those who had two or more high-fructose beverages had a 97 percent higher risk.

In New Zealand, the Maori people rarely encountered gout. Now, ten to fifteen percent of their population has gout symptoms in their lifetime. Seafood seems to be the major trigger for these Pacific islanders; however, they have always eaten a lot of seafood. These people eat fifty times more sugar and fructose (much like typical Americans) than they did 100 years ago.

While high-fructose corn syrup is an obvious problem for your health, you have to be aware of other and natural forms of fructose. Fructose is a sugar molecule found in corn, fruits, agave, and honey, and food or drinks created from them, including fruit juices or food sweetened with agave, honey, or high-fructose corn syrup.

Poor Oxalate Metabolism

Poor oxalate metabolism is another potential cause of gout. Oxalate is a naturally occurring molecule found in fruits, vegetables, nuts, seeds, grains, and legumes. High-oxalate foods include berries, kiwis, purple grapes, figs, potatoes, beets, spinach, okras spinach, rhubarb, Swiss chard, peanuts, soy, cashews, almonds, bran flakes, wheat germs, tea, cacao, and chocolate.

Too much oxalate may cause kidney stones and kidney issues may increase the risk of gout). According to a 2009 study published in Urology Research comparing 100 patients with uric acid stones and gout, 43 patients with gout, 100 patients without gout, and 30 control subjects, there is a relationship between oxalate stone formation and gout.

Certain Medications

Certain medications may also cause gout. According to the American College of Rheumatology, certain diuretics or water pills, including hydrochlorothiazide (Hydro-D and Esidrix) and Lasix, low-dose aspirin intake, and certain immunosuppressants used in organ transplants, including tacrolimus (Prograf) and cyclosporine (Sandimmune and Neoral) may raise uric acid levels and cause gout.

If you are taking any of these medications and experiencing gout, talk to your healthcare professional to check for alternative options and solutions.

2.3   BEST LAB TESTS FOR GOT

Lab tests can help to identify the underlying causes of your gout and also understand your risk factors of developing gout. Lab testing can also help your healthcare provider to create the best, personalized treatment plan to reduce your symptoms of gout, lower your risk of developing gout, and improve your overall health.

I recommend working with a functional health doctor. They are not only able to recommend an array of testing that may not be used at your regular doctor's office but can also help to create a personalized treatment plan focusing on natural support strategies that support your health. There are a variety of lab tests that I recommend.

Uric Acid Levels

Uric acid is created in your body by breaking down purine. Gout is caused by the buildup of uric acid in your body, hence testing your uric acid levels is the first important step and measure to look at your risks of gout.

Uric acid tests are simple urine or blood tests that can help to diagnose gout, determine your risk of gout, and help to monitor gout. Normal uric acid levels are between 3 and 5.5 mg/dL.

Serum Ferritin

A serum ferritin test is a simple test that checks the level of ferritin, a blood cell protein that stores iron, in our body. According to a 2018 study published in

Arthritis Research and Therapy, high ferritin levels may increase your risk of gout.

Low ferritin may also indicate anemia, while high ferritin levels may lead to inflammation, liver disease, autoimmune conditions, and cancer. The optimal range is 30 to 400 and the optimal range is 50 to 150 for females and 75 to 150 for males.

Fasting Insulin

Since insulin resistance and poor blood sugar levels are one of the main causes of gout, it is important to test your fasting insulin levels. Both high or low insulin levels can cause an issue.

High insulin levels are a sign of insulin resistance, prediabetes, diabetes, and metabolic syndrome, which can all lead to inflammation, gout, and other health issues such as hypertension. The clinical range for fasting insulin is between 2.6 and 24.9 uIU/ml and the optimal range is between 1.0 and 5.0 uIU/ml.

HbA1C

Hemoglobin A1C or HbA1c gives the average amount of glucose in the blood, or blood sugar, over the past 3 months. This test is another good indication of poor blood sugar levels, one of the top causes of gout. A high HbA1c is an indication of high levels of advanced glycation end-products (AGE's) that damage proteins and tissues in the body including the red blood cells.

Red blood cells are constantly forming and dying and generally live for about three months, hence this test is a good indication of your blood sugar levels for that period. This is a great test for prediabetes and diabetes, both of which increase your risks of gout. Poor levels of HbA1c also indicate inflammation in the body. The clinical range is between 4.8 and 5.6, but the optimal range is 4.5 to 5.2.

Red Blood Cell Width

The Red Blood Cell Distribution Width (RDW) is a great test to see if there is inflammation in your blood. According to a 2014 study published in Science Reports, there is a correlation between your RDW and uric acid levels.

As you know, elevated uric acid levels can result in gout. Your RDW levels may also indicate a risk for other health issues. The clinical range is between 12.3 and 15.4 percent and the optimal range is 11.7 and 15 percent.

Hs-CRP

C-Reactive Protein (CRP), is a blood test that assesses your inflammation levels. Since gout is characterized by joint inflammation and inflammation is a common underlying cause of most health conditions, it's important to measure your inflammation levels.

CRP is a protein produced by your liver. Increased and decreased levels mean inflammation or trauma that may increase your risk of inflammatory, chronic, and other health issues, including gout and causes of gout. The clinical range is between 0 to 3 mg/L and the optimal range for CRP is between 0 and 2 mg/L.

Oxalate Levels

Checking your oxalate levels is important, since elevated oxalate levels may increase your risk of gout. High levels of oxalate may also indicate an increased risk of developing kidney stones. Normal levels are less than 45 milligrams per day.

To test your oxalate levels, I recommend a Comprehensive Organic Acid Test. This is a simple urine test that looks at complex biomarkers from various metabolic pathways. These biomarkers give an overview of several major systems in the body and an analysis of nutritional deficiencies in the body.

2.4 GOUT TREATMENT

The good news about gout is that you can control it. Medicines help in two ways: They reduce pain during an attack and can reduce the uric acid buildup that causes the condition.

When uric acid builds up in your body, it can form crystals that irritate your joints.

Gout is a type of inflammatory arthritis. An attack may come after an illness or injury. The first sign is often pain in the big toe. It usually affects one joint at a time, but gout can spread to other joints and leave them looking red and swollen.

Talk to Your Doctor About Gout Treatment

The pain from a gout attack usually gets better in 3 to 10 days. But you'll feel better faster with gout treatment. If you think you might have it, contact your doctor. An exam and tests will show if it's gout or something else, like an infection.

Talk with your doctor about the best medicines for you. The type will depend on how well your kidneys work, the possible side effects, and other health issues.

Gout Treatment

Medicines to treat gout center on easing pain and inflammation during a gout attack and lowering uric acid levels in your blood to help avoid future gout-related health problems.

Immediate gout pain relief

NSAIDs offer quick pain relief by helping to lower pain and swelling in the joints during a gout attack. Popular OTC gout treatments are ibuprofen and naproxen. If you take NSAIDs in the first 24 hours, it can help shorten the attack. Other ways to ease pain include ice, rest, and raising the joint. Between gout attacks, you can also take a warm shower and apply heat with a hot water bottle or heating pad.

Gout medications

Your doctor may suggest one of these medicines that you can't get over the counter:

Medicines to ease gout pain and inflammation

- Colchicine (Colcrys, Gloperba, Mitigare) reduces inflammation.
- Indomethacin (Indocin, Tivorbex) is a stronger NSAID pain reliever.
- Steroids (also called corticosteroids) fight inflammation.

Medicines to avoid gout flares and further gout-related health problems

- Allopurinol (Aloprim, Zyloprim) reduces uric acid production.

- Febuxostat (Uloric) reduces uric acid production.

- Lesinurad (Zurampic) helps your body get rid of uric acid when you pee.

- Pegloticase (Krystexxa) breaks down uric acid.

- Probenecid helps the kidneys excrete uric acid from your body.

Gout creams

Creams and gels applied to the skin are another type of gout treatment. Products such as diclofenac (Voltaren) and Gout Buster work by lowering inflammation, swelling, stiffness, and joint pain.

Natural gout treatments

Certain foods and supplements could help to treat gout, including:

- Cherries. Antioxidants called anthocyanins found in the pigment of cherries may help ward off and treat gout by lowering uric acid levels. Studies show concentrated forms of cherries, such as juice, extracts, and supplements, show the most health benefits.
- Bromelain. You'll find this group of enzymes in the fruit and stem of a pineapple. It could ease the pain and swelling of gout and other types of arthritis.
- Vitamin C. Studies show vitamin C can lower uric acid levels in people living with gout and even prevent the illness. You can boost your vitamin C levels with foods like citrus fruit,

peppers, broccoli, and brussels sprouts, or with a supplement.

Talk to your doctor before taking a supplement as part of your gout treatment plan.

Gout Prevention

Along with medicine, your doctor may suggest gout self-care lifestyle changes to prevent another attack:

Exercise and a balanced diet to control your weight Staying hydrated by drinking lots of water

Gout diet

What you eat and drink could play a role in gout attacks.

Food and drinks to avoid:

- Sugary drinks

- Excessive alcohol use, especially beer

- Meat with high purine levels, especially liver, kidney, and sweetbreads

What to eat and drink:

- Fruits, vegetables, and whole grains, which are sources of complex carbs

- Lean meat and poultry, low-fat dairy, and lentils for protein

- Coffee, which may lower your chances of getting gout

- Moderate portions of fish

Gout triggers

High levels of uric acid can trigger gout or a gout attack. Here are some things that may raise your uric acid levels:

- Extra pounds. Your body makes more uric acid, and your kidneys have trouble getting rid of it when you're overweight.

- Medical conditions. Your odds of getting gout rise when you have certain health conditions like untreated high blood pressure, diabetes, obesity, metabolic syndrome, heart disease, and kidney disease.

- Certain medicines. Medicines you take to lower high blood pressure, including thiazide diuretics, ACE inhibitors, and beta blockers, can raise uric acid levels. Low-dose aspirin and antirejection drugs taken after an organ transplant may have the same effect.

- Surgery or trauma. A recent surgery, trauma, or vaccine can trigger a gout attack or flare.

3   Useful Vitamins and Supplements to Manage Gout

Studies have shown that nutrition and nutritional behaviors have a major role in the development of gout. Some relevant factors that affect health include body mass index, excessive intake of alcohol, meat, fruit juices, and soft drinks, which can increase the risk of gout or cause flare-ups in some cases. Consumption of dairy products and coffee can decrease the risk of gout as they help in the excretion of uric acid.

A 2014 study reported the use of dietary supplements mainly including amino acids, antioxidants, essential minerals, polyunsaturated fatty acids, prebiotic agents, probiotic agents, and vitamins. It concluded that there was a reduction in the frequency of gouty attacks and adverse event-related trial withdrawal was also reduced.

Nutritional supplements can help manage gout and reduce flare-ups as certain supplements can help fight off the inflammation, reduce serum uric acid levels in the body, and can boost the immune system.

Here are some of the best vitamins and supplements to manage gout.

Vitamin C

Vitamin C is known for its antioxidant properties and is considered one of the best vitamins and supplements to manage gout. It can reduce cellular damage by neutralizing free radicals and helps keep tissues healthy. It can also help increase the excretion of excess uric acid by stimulating the kidneys and thus help reduce serum uric acid levels.

In a 2005 study, it was concluded that supplementation with 500 mg/day of vitamin C for 2 months reduced serum uric acid. It suggested that vitamin C may be beneficial in the prevention and management of gout.

A 2009 study reported that higher vitamin C intake was linked with a lower risk of gout and that vitamin C supplementation can help in the prevention of gout. It showed up to 45% lower risk at the top vitamin C intake category of 1500 mg or more.

A 2011 study concluded that vitamin C supplementation significantly lowered serum uric acid levels.

Vitamin D

Vitamin D is a fat-soluble vitamin obtained from food, sun exposure, and supplements and serum levels of its form 25-hydroxyvitamin D (25(OH) D) are the best indicators of health. Several studies have shown that vitamin D deficiency increases various health risks and is also one of the best vitamins and supplements to manage gout. It can activate the parathyroid to induce the release of parathyroid hormone that can increase the serum uric acid levels.

A 2020 study reported a lower risk of hyperuricemia with higher serum 25(OH) D, dietary vitamin D intake, and total vitamin D intake and no association between supplemental vitamin D intake and the risk of HU in women among US adults.

A 2021 study done on patients with diabetes and hyperuricemia concluded that vitamin D supplementation lowers serum uric acid in prediabetic patients with hyperuricemia. Thus supplementation may be considered to help alleviate hyperuricemia in these patients.

Skim Milk Powder

Some studies have suggested the use of skim milk powder as it can help reduce the symptoms of gout. This too has found its way to the list of vitamins and supplements to manage gout.

A 2012 study was conducted for 3 months on milk products for the prevention of gout flares. It was the first reported trial of dietary intervention in patients with gout. It concluded that skim milk powder enriched with glycomacropeptide (GMP) and G600 milk fat extract (G600) may reduce the frequency of gouty flare-ups.

Turmeric

Turmeric is not just a popular spice and home remedy but also an important anti-bacterial, anti-septic and anti-inflammatory agent. It is believed to reduce inflammation and help reduce inflammatory arthritis like gout, by also reducing serum uric acid levels, thus considered one of the best supplements to manage gout.

Turmeric, with its active ingredient curcumin, helps control inflammation and pain for ages. It has been used in combination with other nutraceuticals to treat acute and chronic osteoarthritis pain. Recently, the use of turmeric, turmeric extract, or curcuminoids for musculoskeletal pain, has been more popularized.

A 2019 study that used turmeric nanoparticles (T-NPs) to treat gout reported that the uric acid levels were significantly reduced after the treatment and that these can prove to be an efficient antigout agent with minimal toxicities.

Another study concluded that the administration of curcumin could effectively alleviate inflammation caused by monosodium urate (MSU) in gouty arthritis. Thus curcumin therapy can be helpful in the prevention of acute episodes of gout.

Fish Oils

Fish oil supplements contain omega-3-fatty acids, which have anti-inflammatory properties.

However, considering the purine levels, choosing the right type of supplement is important. Studies have shown that when dietary omega-3-PUFA rich fish consumption, adjusted for total purine intake was linked with a lower risk of recurrent gout flares as compared to supplementation alone or taken in a self-directed manner.12 Hence, specific sources and adequate doses of fish oils are required to prevent gout flare-ups.

A 2018 study reported that omega-3-carboxylic acids have anti-inflammatory effects and could be beneficial in the prevention and treatment of crystal arthritis by controlling inflammation.

Bromelain

Bromelain is an enzyme naturally present in Bromelain and is known to have anti-inflammatory properties. It is popularly used in treating people with arthritis, and gout as it helps reduce muscle soreness, pain, and joint swelling.

It is also well-recognized for its antithrombotic and fibrinolytic effects, anticancer activity, and immunomodulatory effects, apart from being a wound healing and circulatory improvement agent.

Ginger

Ginger is known for its medicinal properties and is one of the best supplements to manage gout. Studies have shown its effectiveness as an anti-inflammatory agent that helps control several inflammatory conditions apart from being a popular home remedy for cold, cough, and digestive troubles.

A 2013 study says shagaol, present in ginger has strong anti-inflammatory and antioxidant effects, which can be used to manage gout.

Coffee

A 2016 study reported its results on the effects of consumption of coffee on serum uric acid. It showed that coffee intake of 1 cup/day or more was significantly associated with a reduced risk of gout. It concluded that moderate coffee intake may help primary prevention of hyperuricemia and gout in both genders.

Uric Acid is an end product of purines and damaged or dead cells. It is synthesized in the liver and the intestines. The dead or damaged cells have nucleic acids, guanine, and adenine which degrade and form uric acid. An elevated level of uric acid in the body is a causative agent for various pathological conditions of which the most common is gout. It is also responsible for causing inflammatory arthritis and aids in progression of metabolic syndrome.

All this said, uric acid is the best antioxidant that is naturally available in the body. It helps in protecting the body against various infectious and even neurological conditions. Studies also suggest that uric acid prevents the body from various blood borne diseases although this property of uric acid is still being researched.

When the levels of uric acid are extremely high, they form into crystals and settle in the joints. This results in extreme pain and swelling of the joints. This in medical terms is called gout. Majority of people prefer to treat gout with medical intervention even though lifestyle modifications and dietary changes are also quite effective.

Lowering uric acid levels does wonders for people suffering from gout and other arthritic conditions. This article highlights some of the natural ways to lower uric acid levels in the body.

Restricted intake of Purine Rich Foods: As stated above, purines is one of the ingredients of uric acid. There are many foods which have purines in abundance. Thus identifying and restricting them is the way to go in lowering uric acid levels naturally. Some of the food products that are high on purines include fishes like tuna and sardines.

Red meat, bacon, and some dairy products are also high on purines and aid in elevating the levels of uric acid in the body. Ham and beef is yet another food that is high on purines and should be restricted if not avoided completely. Seafood like lobster and crab are also extremely high on purines.

Medications: There are certain medications which also increase uric acid levels in the body. These medications include diuretics like Lasix, aspirin at a low dose, and immunosuppressants which are normally given before and after a transplant. If an individual has elevated uric acid levels and is on some of these medications then a consultation with a physician is required to change the medication or adjust the dosage.

Healthy Body Weight: Maintaining a healthy body weight is also essential for lowering uric acid levels naturally. If an individual is overweight and obese then shedding off extra weight through healthy means is the need of the hour. Having a close to ideal body weight not only keeps a tab on the uric acid levels but also calm down arthritis and gout flares.

Obesity is a big risk factor for conditions like gout and arthritis. In the same way, if an individual has rapid decline in weight then also the levels of uric acid increase. Thus care should be taken to neither gain too much weight nor lose too much of it. Exercising, eating a balanced and healthy diet, and avoiding saturated fats is the best way to maintain a healthy weight and reduce uric acid level naturally.

Alcohol and Soda Avoidance: Both alcohol and sugary drinks increase uric acid levels if taken in excess. This increases the risk of the individual developing gout. Additionally, these drinks also add unnecessary calories and aid in weight gain. Thus it is important to drink alcohol or sugary drinks in moderation or completely stay off of it if possible to control uric acid levels.

Coffee: There has been some research data available that suggests that people who have a habit of drinking coffee are less likely to develop a condition like gout. This data comes from a study done in 2010 where a nurses' health study was conducted.

It showed that females who consumed about 3 cups of coffee every day had about a 20% decrease in the risk of developing gout when compared to females who did not drink coffee. Similarly females who drank more than 4 cups had a staggering 50% less risk of developing gout than females who did not drink coffee.

Cherries: Research has shown that cherries can reduce the risk of gout even in people who have had a history of this condition. It does this by lowering the uric acid levels naturally. A study done in 2012 in people with gout found out eating cherries for just a couple of days decreased the chances of a gouty flare by almost 35%. This percentage was maintained even with presence of risk factors like age, gender, and use of alcohol.

3.2 AMAZING HOME REMEDIES TO REDUCE URIC ACID

Home remedies have been found to be especially beneficial in reducing uric acid levels in blood. Purines content in food is metabolized to uric acid. Excessive intake of purine containing food causes increased level of uric acid. Excess amount of uric acid is changed to urate. Urate crystal deposits causes gout. It is extremely important to maintain lower level of blood uric acid level to prevent gout. Most of blood uric acid 2/3rd is excreted in kidney and remaining is removed by liver and discharged in to intestine.

Normal Level of Uric Acid

Range is wide for male and female. It is recommended to maintain level below 6 mg / dl in male patient suffering with gout1 and less than 5.5 mg /dl in female patient suffering with gout.

- Female- 3 to 5.7 mg/dl
- Male- Range of 4 to 7 mg/dl is considered normal.

Causes of Excessive Uric Acid in Blood

Higher uric acid concentration in blood is observed in individual suffering with following genetic disorder, diseases, taking medications and consuming food that contains higher quantity of purine.

Metabolic Disorder-

- Alcoholism
- Diuretics

- Diseases-

- Hypothyroidism

- Kidney diseases

- Genetic Disorder

- Genetic disease

- Obesity

- Psoriasis

- Immune Suppression

- Corticosteroids

- Chemotherapy

Vitamin Deficiency

- Niacin deficiency

- Vitamin B3

- Purine-rich Diet

- Sardines

- Dried Beans

- Mushroom

- Liver in diet

- Peas

Not only can they help in reducing and controlling uric acid in mild cases but can also control in advanced cases as well by combining this method with other medications.

So, here are some things that are readily available in most of the food lover's kitchen and can work wonders in reducing high uric acid in our body. Let us start with the most obvious one-

Water

Who knew that the plain old H_2O can be so miraculous? But it is true, drinking ten to twelve glasses of water per day can not only make your skin healthy and glowy but can also stimulate your kidney to excrete uric acid by diluting it. Thus, it reduces uric acid level in blood.

Cherries and Berries

If you want to reduce your uric acid level through home remedies, cherries are your new best friends. Eat fresh cherries, canned cherries, cherry extract and drink cherry juice, in fact, go all out on cherries. Not only this but other dark berries can also help you in reducing uric acid levels.

Olive Oil

It contains Vitamin E, antioxidants as well as monounsaturated fatty acids which do not get destroyed when heated. All these things make it an excellent home remedy to help reduce uric acid level in blood.

Lemon Juice

Lemon juice contains Vitamin C which helps in reducing uric acid. It also, shockingly enough, produces alkalinity and as such helps in neutralizing uric acid. It is, therefore, an excellent home remedy to reduce uric acid in the body.

Baking Soda

It can not only cleanse your utensils but also your body by maintaining the alkalinity of body and helping in excretion of uric acid by making it more soluble. Wonderful home remedy for reducing uric acid; wouldn't you say? Just mix half teaspoon of baking soda in a glass of water and drink it up!

Apple Cider Vinegar

One teaspoon of this in a glass of water can help enormously in eliminating uric acid from the body as it contains malic acid which helps in breakdown and excretion of uric acid. It is an excellent home remedy for cleansing, detoxifying and reducing uric acid in our body.

Potassium-Rich Diet

Potassium is present naturally in various fruits and vegetables in the form of potassium malate and potassium citrate which helps in neutralizing uric acid and its subsequent elimination from the body, thus reducing its levels in the blood.

Avocado, bananas, apricots, dates, figs, kiwis, mangoes, oranges, coconut water, carrots, squash, beets, artichokes, cantaloupes, tomatoes etc. are some of the foods rich in potassium.

Cream of Tartar

Potassium Hydrogen Tartrate, commonly known as cream of tartar, helps in increasing the alkalinity of urine as well as blood. It is a very good home remedy for reducing uric acid. Just dissolve half teaspoon of cream of tartar in a glass of water and well; cheers!

Celery Seeds

Eating celery seeds can be useful home remedy to reduce uric acid level in body as well as in gout and arthritis. It can be taken as fresh or dried seeds or it is also available in the form of capsules and as celery seed extract, so you can choose any of those options.

Stinging Nettle

It is an herb that can cleanse the body of harmful metabolic wastes. It affects lymphatic system, promoting the excretion of waste including uric acid through kidneys. Simmer the leaves in boiling water for ten minutes and drink as tea. You can also add some honey to it.

Sea Salt

If you want to reduce your uric acid level, say no to salts. Avoid foods rich in salt as well as packaged foods that have a high quantity of sodium in it. Instead of regular table salt, use sea salt only sparingly. Just follow the low salt rule for a few weeks and you will notice that your taste buds have adapted and you can no longer tell the difference in taste.

Soaking in Hot Water

In acute cases, where high uric acid has developed into arthritic gout, soaking hands and feet in hot water can help in dissolving uric acid crystals and thus helps in reducing uric acid level naturally at home.

Some other home remedies to reduce the level of uric acid in our body involves using turmeric, honey, garlic, ginger etc.

So, these were some of the "minimal pain, huge gain" type of home remedies to help you in reducing your uric acid level and bouncing you back to health and happiness.

4   Overview of Purine

So what is the official purine definition in biology? Purines are a type of organic compound found in a variety of different foods, but they can also be produced naturally by the body. Chemically speaking, purines and pyrimidines form the building blocks of DNA and play a key role in maintaining overall health.

However, purine bases are also broken down into uric acid, which can form crystals that accumulate in the joints and contribute to gout, a type of arthritis that causes severe pain and inflammation. For this reason, a low-purine diet for gout is often recommended to help prevent uric acid from building up in the blood.

A gout diet menu is also sometimes recommended for those with kidney stones caused by the build-up of uric acid.

4.1   WHAT IS A LOW-PURINE DIET?

A low-purine diet involves reducing your intake of certain foods to decrease the purine metabolism pathways, which are responsible for converting purines into uric acid.

Healthy whole foods like fruits, veggies, nuts, seeds and legumes are all encouraged as part of the diet while ingredients like red meat, seafood, wild game and organ meats should be consumed only in moderation.

Foods high in fructose, which is a type of simple sugar, should also be limited. Fructose is broken down into purine, which can increase levels of uric acid in the body. Although fructose is found naturally in fruits, these foods are also high in fiber, vitamins and minerals that can offset any negative effects.

Conversely, soft drinks, fruit juice and processed foods all typically contain a concentrated amount of fructose and should be limited on a low-purine diet.

Low-purine diets are recommended for those with gout or certain types of kidney stones to prevent flare-ups and minimize symptoms. A low-purine diet for dogs is also sometimes recommended to prevent uric acid kidney stones from forming in certain breeds who may be more susceptible.

4.2 LOW PURINE BENEFITS

Prevents Gout Flare-Ups

Gout is a type of arthritis that is characterized by swelling, pain and redness in the joints. Fortunately, making just a few minor modifications to your diet can help prevent flare-ups and reduce gout symptoms.

For instance, according to a 2012 study out of Boston, frequent consumption of purine-rich foods increased the risk of recurrent gout attacks by nearly fivefold among those with gout. Another study published in Asia Pacific Journal of Clinical Nutrition reported that regular intake of purine-rich foods like red meat, seafood and alcohol was tied to higher levels of uric acid in the blood.

Protects Against Kidney Stones

Certain types of kidney stones are caused by high levels of uric acid. Increased excretion of uric acid through the urine causes the urine to become more acidic, making it easier for uric acid stones to form and causing symptoms like lower back pain, nausea, vomiting, fever, chills and blood in the urine.

In one study out of Iran, increased consumption of purine-rich foods was linked to a higher risk of developing kidney stones. A 2013 review published by the Universidade Federal de São Paulo also noted that reducing consumption of animal protein could help decrease purine intake and uric acid excretion to prevent kidney stones.

Prioritizes Nutrient-Dense Foods

Nutritious ingredients like fruits, veggies, nuts, seeds and legumes are all encouraged as part of a low-purine diet plan. Meanwhile, other foods like red meat, processed meat and alcohol should all be limited on the diet.

Not only can help ensure that you're getting the nutrients that you need to support better health, but it can also protect against nutritional deficiencies as well as symptoms like fatigue, hair loss, weakness and constipation.

4.3   FOODS TO EAT

A typical low-purine foods chart is very balanced and contains an array of healthy ingredients, including fruits, veggies, nuts, seeds and legumes.

Here are a few of the foods that can be enjoyed as part of a low-purine diet plan:

- Fruits: apples, oranges, bananas, pears, peaches, melons, berries
- Vegetables: broccoli, kale, potatoes, zucchini, carrots, garlic, onions, Brussels sprouts
- Nuts: almonds, walnuts, macadamia nuts, pistachios, cashews
- Seeds: chia seeds, flax seeds, hemp seeds, pumpkin seeds, sunflower seeds
- Legumes: beans, peas, lentils, chickpeas, peanuts
- Whole grains: oats, millet, quinoa, couscous, farro, buckwheat, barley
- Dairy products: milk, yogurt, cheese, kefir, grass-fed butter
- Eggs: egg yolks and whites

- Herbs and spices: cinnamon, black pepper, turmeric, ginger, coriander, oregano, basil
- Beverages: water, tea, coffee

Foods to Avoid

Processed meat, fish and organ meats are all examples of high-purine foods that should be limited on a low-purine diet. Here are some of the key purine-rich foods that you should consume in moderation:

- Organ meats: kidneys, tripe, liver, sweetbread, tongue
- Seafood: anchovies, trout, haddock, herring, sardines, tuna, mackerel
- Red meat: beef, lamb, pork
- Wild game: venison, duck, veal, elk

- Processed meat: ham, hot dogs, salami, bologna, jerky

- Refined carbohydrates: baked goods, cookies, crackers, white bread, pasta

- Alcohol: beer, wine, liquor

- Added sugar: high-fructose corn syrup, agave syrup, honey

- Sugar-sweetened beverages: soda, fruit juice, sports drinks, sweet tea

Some other plant-based ingredients may also contain purines as well, including spinach, cauliflower, mushrooms and dried beans and peas. However, research generally shows that these high-purine vegetables don't have the same impact on uric acid levels as animal-based products and can be included in moderation as part of a low-purine diet menu.

Tips for Following the Diet

Following a low-purine diet doesn't have to be difficult. In fact, it simply involves enjoying a variety of nutrient-rich foods that are low in purines such as fruits, veggies, nuts and seeds while also limiting your consumption of organ meats, processed meat, wild game and certain types of seafood.

Reducing your intake of alcohol can also help decrease purine consumption and keep uric acid levels low. According to one study in Clinical Rheumatology, increased alcohol consumption was associated with a higher risk of gout. However, the type of alcohol may also make a difference. In fact, one study noted that intake of beer and spirits was tied to an increased risk of gout whereas moderate consumption of wine was not.

It's also important to stay hydrated and drink plenty of water during the day, which can help promote the excretion of uric acid through the urine to prevent it from building up in the body. Be sure to always keep a glass of water on hand or try setting a timer with reminders to drink more water throughout the day.

There are plenty of low-purine recipes available online, which make it easy to find healthy meals to add to your routine. Here are a few simple recipes to help get you started:

- Tropical Acai Bowl
- Hearty Spaghetti Squash Casserole
- Tomato Basil Calzone
- Eggplant Rollatini
- Thai Curry Kelp Noodles

4.4 RISKS AND SIDE EFFECTS

Although the low-purine diet is often recommended to minimize gout attacks and reduce symptoms, other medications and treatment methods may also be necessary. For example, anti-inflammatory medications are often prescribed to relieve symptoms during a flare-up and other types medications are also sometimes used to decrease uric acid production in the body.

Additionally, keep in mind that a low-purine diet may not aid in the prevention of all types of kidney stones. In fact, if you have calcium oxalate, cystine or struvite kidney stones, other dietary modifications, lifestyle changes and treatment methods may be required.

Because many of the animal proteins high in purines are also rich in other important nutrients like zinc, iron and omega-3 fatty acids, it's also crucial to ensure that you're getting these vitamins and minerals from other sources in your diet.

Although you can enjoy nutrient-rich foods like beef and seafood in moderation as part of a low-purine diet, you should also consume a variety of other healthy foods like vegetables, beans, nuts and seeds to help fill in any gaps in your diet.

5.1   CURRIED CARROT, POTATO, AND GINGER SOUP

Ingredients

2 Teaspoons of Canola Oil

1 Tablespoon of Sugar

½ Cup of Shallots

3 Cups of Sweet Potato (peeled)

1 Tablespoon of Ginger

2 Teaspoons of Curry Powder

3 Cups of Chicken Broth

Salt and Pepper

Directions

Begin by heating the oil in a pan over a medium flame

Place shallots into the pan and sauté for three minutes

Add carrots, ginger, potato, and curry and mix together; cook this mixture for 2 minutes

Pour in broth and bring it to a bowl

Place a lid over the bowl, lower the heat, and allow the mixture to simmer for twenty minutes

Add salt and pepper to taste

Pour the resulting soup into a bowl and allow it to cool before serving

5.2 WALDORF SALAD

Ingredients

2 Tablespoons of Mayonnaise

1 Tablespoon of Lemon Juice

8 Leaves of Lettuce

¼ Cup of Celery

¼ Cup of Walnuts

1 Cup of Grapes

2 Apples

1/3 Cup of Cranberries (dried)

Directions

Mix the lemon juice, mayonnaise, grapes, apples, and cranberries together in a bowl

Add celery and walnuts and mix thoroughly again

Pour mixture over lettuce leaves

Either serve immediately or refrigerate for up to two hours

5.3   AMARANTH PORRIDGE

Ingredients

2/3 cups of Amaranth Grain

2 Cups of Water

1 Tablespoon of Honey

¼ Hemp of Pumpkin Seeds

½ Cup of Blueberries

1 Pear (chopped)

Directions

Mix the amaranth and water together in a skillet

Place the skillet over a medium to high flame and allow it to boil before bringing it back to a low flame

Allow the mixture to simmer for twenty five minutes and stir periodically

Remove the mixture from the flame and add the rest of the ingredients except for the pear and blueberries

Pour the resulting porridge into bowls and add the blueberries and pear

Serve

5.4 Kale Chips

Ingredients

2 Bunches of Washed Kale

1 Cup of Sweet Potato (grated)

1 Tablespoon of Honey

2 Tablespoon of Yeast

1 Lemon

1 Cup of Cashews

2 Tablespoon of Water

Salt and Pepper

Directions

Set your oven to one hundred and fifty degrees
Fahrenheit

Set the kale into a bowl

Mix the rest of the ingredients together in a blender
and process it until it has become smooth

Pour the processed ingredients over the kale and
mix together

Place what you have prepared so far on parchment
paper and set it in the oven

Keep the mixture in the oven for two hours

Remove from oven and store in a container until
serving

5.5   BEET SALAD

Ingredients

1 Beet (grated)

1 Carrot (grated)

1 Apple

2 Tablespoons of Lemon Juice

2 Tablespoons of Pumpkin Seed Oil

1 Tablespoon of Almonds

4 Cups of Lettuce

Directions

Mix all of the ingredients, except for the lettuce, in a bowl

Place one cup of lettuce over every plate, for four plates total

Pour the mixed ingredients over the lettuce plates and serve

5.6   Kiwi Kale Smoothie

Ingredients

2 Kiwifruits

2 Cups of Kale

5 Ounces of Water

1 Mango

1 Orange

Directions

Put all of the ingredients together in a blender and process until it has mix together into a smoothie

Pour into a glass and serve

5.7   Raw Pad Thai

Ingredients

1 Zucchini

1 Green Onion

1 Carrot

½ Cup of Bean Sprouts

½ Cup of Cauliflower Florets

½ Cup of Cabbage

2 Tablespoons of Tahini (for sauce)

2 Tablespoons of Almond Butter (for sauce)

1 Tablespoon of Honey (for sauce)

1 Tablespoon of Tamari (for sauce)

1 Tablespoon of Lemon Juice (for sauce)

½ Teaspoon of Ginger Root (for sauce)

½ Teaspoon of Garlic (for sauce)

Direction

Run the zucchini and the carrots through a vegetable peeler to make noodles

Place the noodles into a bowl and top them off with the rest of the vegetables

Take all of the sauce ingredients and mix together in a bowl; whisk until thick

Pour the completed sauce over the vegetables and mix them thoroughly together; the sauce should thin out

Pour into bowls and serve

5.8 Key Lime Pie

Ingredients

1 Cup of Shredded Coconut (for crust)

1 Cup of Walnuts (for crust)

½ Cup of Pitted Dates (for crust)

1/4 Teaspoon of Salt (for crust)

3 Avocados (for filling)

½ Cup of Honey (for filling)

1 Teaspoon of Lime Juice (for filling)

3 Tablespoon of Lime Juice (for filling)

Kiwi Slices as Desired

Directions

Mix the walnuts, coconuts, and salt together and process until grounded

Add dates and process again

Press the mixture into the sides of a pie plate with the aid of a spoon to make the crust

Freeze the crust for 15 minutes

Place all of the ingredients for the filling in a processer and process until they have smoothed

Pour the filling into the crust, and add kiwi slices as desired

Place in the refrigerator for twenty minutes

Serve

5.9 MELON MANGO SMOOTHIE

Ingredients

2 Cups of Cantaloupe

2 Leaves of Chard

6 Strawberries

2 Mangoes

5 Ounces of Water

1 Stalk of Celery

2 Cups of Spinach

Directions

Pour the water into a blender and add each of the ingredients

Process until it has mixed well into a liquid smoothie form

Pour into a glass and serve

5.10 KALE SALAD

Ingredients

6 Cups of Kale

½ Lemon

1 Pinch of Basil

1 Pinch of Salt

1 Tablespoon of Olive Oil

1 Cucumber

2 Tablespoons of Green Onion

2 Tablespoons of Red Onion

1 Clove of Garlic

¼ Cup of Olives

Directions

Cut the kale into thin strips

Steam the kale strips for 6 minutes

Transfer the steamed kale strips to a bowl

Mix olive oil, salt, basil, and lemon with the kale thoroughly together

Add the rest of the ingredients and mix again

Serve

5.11   PINEAPPLE-GRAPEFRUIT SMOOTHIE

Ingredients

1 Banana (peeled)

5 Ounces of Water

½ Cup of Cilantro

½ Cucumber

1 Cup of Pineapple

½ Grapefruit

Directions

Place all of the ingredients into a blender and process until in smoothie form
Pour into a glass and serve

5.12   CINNAMON BAKED APPLES

Ingredients

½ Cup of Nuts

¼ Cup of Cranberries

4 Apples

¼ Teaspoon of Cloves

½ Teaspoon of Nutmeg

1 Teaspoon of Cinnamon

1 Teaspoon of Ginger Root

2 Dates

1 Cup of Apple Juice

¼ Cup of Honey

Directions

Preheat your oven to 325 degrees Fahrenheit

Mix the cranberries, nuts, ginger root, dates, and spices together in a bowl

Cut out the core from each apple, and then fill up the resulting hole with the mixture

Cover the apples in honey and place on a baking dish

Pour apple juice around and over the apples

Bake for a half hour

Remove from oven and serve

5.13   PINEAPPLE AND CARROT SMOOTHIE

Ingredients

1 Orange

2 Cups of Pineapple

2 Carrots

2 Tablespoons of Chia Seeds

8 Ounces of Water

2 Cups of Spinach

½ Teaspoon of Ginger

Directions

Place all of the ingredients in a blender and process until it has liquefied thoroughly into smoothie form

Pour into a glass and serve

5.14 CHERRY-CINNAMON APPLE BAKE

Ingredients

1 Cup of Cherries

2 Apples

1 Tablespoon of Cinnamon

½ Teaspoon of Nutmeg

3 Tablespoons of Raisins

Directions

Preheat your oven to 375 degrees Fahrenheit

Mix all of the ingredients thoroughly together

Set the mixture on an oven baking dish and bake for
45 minutes

Remove from oven and serve

5.15 WATERMELON-PINEAPPLE JUICE

Ingredients

1/3 Pineapple

2 Slices of Watermelon

1 Inch of Ginger Root

Directions

Cut the core out of the pineapple

Place all of the ingredients into a juicer and process
until in liquefied form

Pour into ice glasses and serve

5.16 GINGER POTATO SOUP

Ingredients:

1 Tablespoon of Olive Oil

2 Sweet Potatoes

1 Clove of Garlic

2 Teaspoon of Ginger

4 Leaves of Mint

1/3 Teaspoon of Turmeric

2 Cups of Vegetable Broth

Directions

Pour the olive oil into a food processor

Peel the sweet potatoes and place them into the processor next

Add garlic gloves, turmeric, mint leaves and ginger next

Process the mixture together

Pour into a pot and set it over a medium flame for

30 Minutes

Serve

5.17 CHICKEN THYME CASSEROLE

Ingredients

1 Cup of Dark Chicken Meat

2 Cups of Brown Rice

½ Cup of Water

½ Cup of Peas

½ Cup of Carrots

2 Teaspoons of Thyme

1 Teaspoon of Celery

Salt and Pepper

Directions:

Brown the pieces of chicken in an oven

Mix brown rice, water, carrots, salt and pepper, celery, thyme, and peas together with the chicken in a pot

Set the bowl over a high flame until it boils

Reduce the flame to low and allow the mixture to simmer for 30 Minutes

Serve

5.18 Avocado Cabbage Rolls

Ingredients

1 Tablespoon of Olive Oil

1 Avocado

1 Tablespoon of Apple Cider Vinegar

1 Head of Cabbage

½ Tablespoon of Chili Powder

1 Small Onion

Directions

Preheat your oven to 425 degrees Fahrenheit

Add 1 tablespoon of olive oil to a skillet

Saute onion in the olive oil for a minute

Add chili powder, apple cider, vinegar, and avocado
and mix

Fill up each cabbage leaf with the mix

Set on baking tray and bake for 12 minutes

Serve

5.19 SPICED ASPARAGUS

Ingredients

12 Asparagus

1 Tablespoon of Olive Oil

1 Cup of bread Crumbs

1 Cup of Parmesan

½ Tablespoon of Jalapeno Powder

Directions

Preheat your oven to 400 degrees Fahrenheit

Mix olive oil, bread crumbs, jalapenos, and parmesan together in a bowl

Place asparagus into the mixture until cover

Set on a baking tray and bake for 20 minutes

Serve

5.20 MORNING PIE

Ingredients

1 Tablespoon of Olive Oil

1 Teaspoon of Garlic

1/3 Cup of Salsa

1 Roll of Biscuit Dough

½ Cup of Cheddar cheese

4 Egg Whites

Directions

Mix garlic, salsa, and egg whites thoroughly together

Cover with pieces of your biscuit dough

Top off with cheese

Cook in a crock pot at medium heat for two hours

Cool and serve

5.21 CINNAMON ROLL

Ingredients

1 Cinnamon Roll

2 Tablespoons of Melted Butter

2 Cups of White Sugar

¾ Tablespoon of Brown Sugar

23/ Cup of Lemon Juice

4 Teaspoons of Cinnamon

1 Cup of Pecan Pieces

Directions

Mix the white sugar and lemon juice together in a bowl

In a second bowl, mix the brown sugar, pecan, and cinnamon

Roll the cinnamon dough into a flat sheet piece and pour melted butter over it

Cook for one hour in a crock pot on high

Remove from crock pot and coat with both sugar mixtures

Cook on high for another half hour

Serve

5.22 TOMATO AND AVOCADO CASSEROLE

Ingredients

Cubed Ciabatta Bread

1 Tablespoon of Olive Oil

1/3 Cup of Scallions

1 Avocado

½ Cup of Tomatoes

3 Leaves of Basil

1 Cup of Mozzarella

Directions

Preheat your oven to 350 degrees Fahrenheit

Mix together olive oil, tomatoes, scallions, basils, and avocado in a bowl

Place the Ciabatta bread in a dish and top with the above mixture and cheese

Bake for 20 minutes

Serve

5.23 CHERRY POLENTA

Ingredients

1 Tablespoon of Butter

Olive Oil as Desired

2 Cups of Polenta

2 Cups of Milk

1 ½ Cup of Cherries

Directions

Mix polenta, butter, olive oil, and milk together and stir

Bring this mixture to a boil over a high flame

Reduce the heat and allow it to simmer for 40 minutes

Add cherries and serve

5.24 ENCHILADAS FRITTATA

Ingredients

6 Egg Whites

Olive Oil as Desired

½ Can of Sodium

1/3 Cup of Salsa

1 Teaspoon of Hot Sauce

2/3 Tablespoon of Chili Powder

1 Teaspoon of Cumin

1 Teaspoon of Celery

1 Package of Cheddar cheese

Directions

Prepare a skillet over a medium heat and melt butter with olive oil

Mix tomatoes, egg whites, salsa, hot sauce, cumin, chili powder, and celery

Top with cheese and cook over skillet for 20 minutes before serving

5.25 ROSEMARY SHELLS

Ingredients

1 Tablespoon of Olive Oil

1 Package of Stuffed Shells

½ Cup of Ricotta Cheese

1 Tablespoon of Rosemary

½ Cup of Tomatoes

Directions

Preheat oven to 400 degrees Fahrenheit

Pour in olive oil into a dish

Place the shells on dish with their open sides up

Mix cheese, tomatoes, and rosemary and pour the mixture into the open shells

Cook for 30 minutes before serving

5.26 Crockpot Macaroni and Cheese

Ingredients

1 Tablespoon of Olive Oil

1 Tablespoon of Butter

1 Teaspoon of Garlic

1 Tablespoon of Sriracha Sauce

1 Teaspoon of Onion Powder

1 Cup of Chicken Bouillon

½ Cup of Milk

8 Ounces of Macaroni

1 Cup of Monterey Jack Cheese

½ Cups of Bread Crumbs

Directions

Mix all of the ingredients except for the macaroni and cheese in a crock pot

Add the macaroni and cheese and stir thoroughly together

Cook over a low heat for an hour and a half before serving

5.27 MARINATED EGGPLANT DISH

Ingredients

1 Tablespoon of Olive Oil

½ Tablespoon of Butter

1 Teaspoon of Worcester Sauce

1/3 Cup of Honey

1/3 Cup of Brown Sugar

1 Teaspoon of Black Pepper

1 Tablespoon of Ginger Powder

1 Onion

1 Cup of Eggplant

Directions

Mix olive oil, honey, sugar, ginger, pepper, and butter in a bag to form a marinade

Place the onion and eggplant in the marinade and set it in a refrigerator for four hours

Remove from refrigerator and simmer over a high flame for 5 minutes before serving

5.28 Avocado Medley

Ingredients

¾ Tablespoon of Olive Oil

1 Cup of Brown Rice

¾ Cup of Water

Garlic to taste

1 Tomato

1 Onion

1 Cup of Egg Plant

1 Avocado

¼ Cup of lemon Juice

1 Tablespoon of Basil

Directions

Pour the olive oil in a pot and warm over a high flame

Saute tomato, eggplants, avocado, and onion in olive oil for 2 minutes

Pour lemon juice, water, rice, and garlic into the mixture and boil while stirring

Reduce heat and allow it to simmer for 25 minutes before serving

5.29 Zucchini Casserole

Ingredients

3 Zucchinis

1 Cup of Mozzarella

1/3 Cup of Olive Oil

½ Tablespoon of Parsley

1 Tablespoon of Rosemary

Directions

Preheat oven to 400 degrees Fahrenheit

Place Zucchini in a bowl, and mix it with the rest of the ingredients

Bake for 20 minutes before serving

5.30 Thyme Stuffed Peppers

Ingredients

2 Bell Peppers

1 Tablespoon of Olive Oil

½ Cup of Rice

1 Can of Tomatoes

1 Cup of Beef Brother

½ Tablespoon of Thyme

½ Cup of Parmesan

Directions

Remove seeds from peppers and place peppers inside a crock pot

Mix rice, broth, tomatoes, and thyme together

Place the mixture into the open peppers and sprinkle with cheese

Cook over a low heat for three hours before serving

5.31 Cucumber Boats

Ingredients

2 Cucumbers

1 Tomato

1 Shallot

1 Tablespoon of Italian Dressing

½ Tablespoon of Chia Seeds

Directions

Preheat oven to 325 Degrees Fahrenheit

Cut the cucumbers in half and lay with the open side up

Mix tomatoes, shallot, dressing, and cheese together and place on the open cucumbers; top with seeds

Bake for 15 Minutes before serving

5.32 ALFREDO, LINGUINE, AND TORTELLINI CASSEROLE

Ingredients

1 Tablespoon of Olive Oil

1 Teaspoon of Garlic

½ Shallot

2 Cups of Cheese Tortellini

1 Cup of Alfredo Sauce

1 Teaspoon of oregano

1 Cup of Italian Cheese

8 Ounces of Linguine

Directions

Preheat Oven to 350 degrees Fahrenheit

Cook Linguine according to instructions on the package

Mix Alfredo sauce, tortellini, oregano, and Italian cheese together

Pour into a dish and bake for 30 minutes

5.33 CORNBREAD CASSEROLE

Ingredients

2 Cups of Green Beans

½ Cup of Corn

½ Cup of Carrots

3 Cups of Cornbread (crumbled)

1 Teaspoon of Sage

½ Teaspoon of Cloves

Directions

Preheat oven to 350 degrees Fahrenheit

Mix butter, beans, corn, carrots, cloves, and sage in
a bowl

Place crumbled cornbread on the bottom of a dish

Place mixture over the cornbread

Cook for 30 Minutes

5.34 GINGER STIR FRY AND COCONUT RICE

Ingredients:

½ Teaspoon of Corn Starch

½ Cloves of Garlic

½ Teaspoon of Ginger Root

2 Teaspoons of Olive Oil

1 Tablespoons of Red Bell Pepper

2 Tablespoons of Carrots

1 Teaspoon of Soy Sauce

Water

½ Tablespoon of Chopped Onion

¼ Cup of Jasmine Rice

¼ Cup of Coconut Milk

¼ Cup of Hot Sauce

Directions

Place rice, coconut milk, and water in a pot and boil over a high flame

Reduce to low heat and allow the mixture to simmer for 15 minutes

Mix corn starch, ginger, garlic, and olive oil together

Add peas, broccoli, carrots, and bell pepper together

Heat olive oil over a medium heat and sauté vegetables for 1 minute

Add salt, ginger, onions, soy sauce, and water; cook for 2 minutes

Please the coconut rice in an eating bowl and top off with the ginger stir fry mix and hot sauce

5.35 BOK CHOY MEDLEY

Ingredients

1 Cup of Rice

1 Tablespoon of Apple Cider Vinegar

1/3 Cup of Honey

½ Teaspoon of Black Pepper

½ Teaspoon of Cayenne Powder

1 Diced Bok Choy

1 Cup of Fajita Peppers

Onions to taste

Directions

Preheat oven to 350 degrees Fahrenheit

Pour rice into a dish and add vinegar and honey

Add bok choy, fajitas, onions, black pepper, and cayenne powder over the rice

Cover up with a foil and cook for a half hour

5.36 Avocado Tacos

Ingredients

Corn Tortillas

1 Avocado

2 Tablespoons of Inions

1/8 Teaspoon of Garlic

1 Teaspoon of Lemon Juice

Olive Oil to Taste

2 Tablespoons of Tomatoes

2 Teaspoons of Cilantro

Salt and Pepper to taste

½ Clove of Garlic

¼ Cup of Black Beans

Directions

Preheat your oven to 325 degrees Fahrenheit

Heat olive oil over a medium flame

Add onions and garlic and cook for 3 minutes

Lower heat and add black beans

Set out tortillas on a baking sheet and heat in oven for 2 minutes

Mix avocado, garlic, lemon juice, salt and pepper, and olive oil in a bowl

Spread this mixture over the tortillas, and add onions and garlic, black beans, and cilantro before serving

5.37 MEX STACKERS

Ingredients

10 Tortilla Shells

2 Cups of Salsa

1/3 Cup of Turmeric Powder

½ Can of Black Beans

1 Package of Mexican Cheese

Directions

Preheat Oven to 350 Degrees Fahrenheit

Mix turmeric powder, black beans, and salsa in a bowl

Cut 3 inch circles out of the tortillas

Add a spoonful of the mixture over each tortilla circle and cover with cheese

Bake for 15 minutes and serve

5.38 QUINOA CHARD PILAF

Ingredients

1 Teaspoon of Olive Oil

1 Tablespoon of Onion

1 Clove of Garlic

¼ Cup of Quinoa

2 Tablespoon of Lentils

½ Cup of Vegetable Broth

¼ Bunch of Swiss Chard

Directions

Heat oil in a pot over a medium flame

Add garlic and onion and stir together; sauté for 5 minutes

Add lentils and quinoa

Pour in broth

Cook for 15 minutes

Remove pot from the flame

Mix chard into the pot and cook for 5 more minutes before serving

5.39 Nacho Muffins

Ingredients

1 Tablespoon of Olive Oil

1 Cup of Tomatoes

2 Scallions

1 Teaspoon of Basil

2 Teaspoons of Chili Powder

3 Ounces of Chicken

1 Cup of Mexican Cheese

Directions

Preheat oven to 350 Degrees Fahrenheit

Mix tortilla chips with olive oil in a processor

Press into molds on a muffin mold tray

Mix tomatoes, spices, scallions, and chicken in a bowl

Pour into the muffin molds

Bake for 30 minutes and serve

5.40 MEDITERRANEAN ZUCCHINI

Ingredients

1 Teaspoon of Olive Oil

2 Tablespoon of Red Bell Pepper

2 Tablespoons of Onion

1 Clove of Garlic

¼ Cup of Tomatoes

¼ Cup of Cannellini Beans

½ Cup of Zucchini

Salt and Pepper to Taste

Water

¼ Cup of Rice

Directions

Pour water and rice into a pot over a high flame and cook until boiling

Reduce heat and allow it to simmer for 15 minutes

Heat olive oil in a saucepan over a medium heat

Add peppers, onions, and garlic, and cook for 5 minutes

Add zucchini, salt and pepper, oregano, and tomatoes and simmer for 20 minutes while stirring

Add beans and continue to cook for 10 minutes

Add in rice and serve

5.41 SPRING ROLLS

Ingredients

6 Rice Paper Wrappers

½ Cup of Carrots

½ Cup of Cucumbers

1 Teaspoon of Vinegar

1 Cup of Avocado

1 Teaspoon of Lemon Juice

½ Tablespoon of Apple Cider Vinegar

Directions

Preheat Oven to 350 Degrees Fahrenheit

Lay out your wraps on the tray

Mix carrots, avocado, cucumber, lemon juice, vinegar, and apple cider vinegar together on a bowl

Add the mixture into each wrapper

Roll up the wrappers

Bake for 30 minutes and serve

5.42 HUMMUS ZEST

Ingredients

2/3 Cup of Chickpeas

½ Tablespoon of Olive Oil

1 Teaspoon of Red Peppers

1 Teaspoon of Oregano

½ Teaspoon of Thyme

Directions

Mix the oil, chickpeas, red pepper flakes, thyme, and oregano in a processor and process it

Store the mixture in a container in the refrigerator for up to three days or serve now

5.43 MAC AND NO CHEESE

Ingredients:

¾ Cup of Macaroni

1 Teaspoon of Olive Oil

1 Clove of Garlic

¼ Cup of Cashews

2 Tablespoons of Onion

2 Tablespoons of Red Peppers

Water

Salt and Pepper to Taste

1 Tablespoon of Lemon Juice

½ Teaspoon of Garlic Powder

½ teaspoon of Onion Powder

Directions

Preheat oven to 350 Degrees Fahrenheit

Boil a pot of salted water

Add pasta to the pot and cook for 10 minutes

Transfer to a baking dish

Heat olive oil in a saucepan and sauté onion and garlic for 4 minutes

Add macaroni and use a food processor to blend cashews, lemon juice, salt and pepper, and water together 1 olive oil, garlic powder, onion powder, and red peppers together

Blend until mixed together

Combine the mixtures with the macaroni and bake for 45 minutes

Cool, add black peppers, and serve

5.44 AVOCADO FRIES

Ingredients

3 Egg Whites

1/3 Cup of Bread Crumbs

½ Cup of Flower

¼ Cup of Parmesan

2 Avocados

Directions

Preheat oven to 425 Degrees Fahrenheit

Mix egg whites together and in a separate bowl mix breadcrumbs, cheese, and flower

Add avocado pieces into the egg mix and the flour mix separately

Place the avocado pieces on a baking tray

Bake for 20 minutes and serve

5.45 POTATO CURRY

Ingredients

1 Teaspoon of Virgin Oil

2 Potatoes

1 Tablespoon of Onion

1 Clove of Garlic

½ Teaspoon of Ground Cumin

½ Teaspoon of Cayenne

2 Teaspoon of Ginger Root

1 Pinch of Salt

1 Tomato

¾ Teaspoon of Curry Powder

¼ Cup of Coconut Milk

Directions

Cut potato into cubes and place cubes in a pot with salt and water

Boil this over a high head, and then reduce heat and simmer for 15 minutes

Heat olive oil in a skillet and sauté garlic and onion for 5 minutes

Season with cumin, curry powder, cayenne pepper, ginger, and salt and pepper

Cook for 2 more minutes

Add beans, tomatoes, and more potatoes and pour in coconut milk

Simmer for 10 minutes and serve

5.46 Chicken-Celery Sticks

Ingredients

4 Stalks of Celery

3 Ounces of Cream Cheese

2 Teaspoons of Basil

1/3 Cup of Chicken Cubes

Directions

Allow your cream cheese to sit for 30 minutes

Cut celery stocks into three pieces

Mix the stalks, basil, chicken cubes, and cream cheese in a bowl

Refrigerate for up to three days or serve now

5.47 Quinoa Chard Pilaf

Ingredients

1 teaspoon of olive oil

1 tablespoon of onions

1 clove of garlic

¼ cup of quinoa

2 tablespoon of lentils

½ cup of vegetable broth

¼ bunch of swiss chard

Directions

Heat the olive oil in a pot of a medium flame

Add onion and garlic and sauté for 5 minutes

Add lentils quinoa, and brother

Cook for 15 minutes

Get rid of head and shred chard into the pot

Cover pot and sit for 5 minutes

Serve

5.48 STUFFED PEPPERS (NO MEAT)

Ingredients

1 Cup of Cauliflower

¾ Tablespoon of Melted Butter

1/3 Tablespoon of Garlic

4 Bell Peppers

½ Cup of Eggplant

1 Teaspoon of Basil

½ Teaspoon of Oregano

Directions

Preheat your oven to 350 Degrees Fahrenheit

Remove seeds from peppers and place in a dish

Process cauliflower, oil, butter, garlic, and puree in a food processor until mashed together

Place this mixture into peppers, and top with eggplant, oregano, basil, and cheese

Bake for 30 minutes and serve

5.49 Veggie and Lentil Bake

Ingredients

½ Cup of Rice

Water

1 Cup of Lentils

1 Teaspoon of Olive Oil

1 Onion

3 Cloves of Garlic

1 Tomato

1/3 Cup of Celery

1 Teaspoon of Basil

1/3 Cup of Zucchini

1/3 Cup of Carrots

1 Can of Tomato

1 Teaspoon of Cumin

½ Teaspoon of Celery

Salt and Pepper

Directions

Preheat your oven to 350 Degrees Fahrenheit

Mix oregano, basil, cumin, celery seeds, and salt and pepper in a bowl

Pour rice and water into a pot over a high flame and boil

Reduce heat and allow it to simmer for 20 minutes

Set lentils in a pot with more water and cook for 15 minutes over a medium to high heat

Heat oil in a skillet over a medium flame and add garlic and onion

Mix tomato, celery, carrots, tomato sauce, and zucchini together

Season with seasoning mix

In a dish, mix lentils, rice, and vegetables

Top off with tomato sauce, and sprinkle on more seasoning

Bake for 30 minutes in your oven

Remove and mix all of the mixtures together and serve

5.50 Grilled Tomato/Balsamic Veggie Dish

Ingredients

1 Teaspoon of Olive Oil

¼ Red Bell Pepper

¼ Zucchini

¼ Eggplant

¼ Sweet Onion

3 Tablespoons of Beans

2 Tomatoes

2 Teaspoons of Vinegar

¼ Cup of Couscous

¼ Cup of Vegetable Stock

Directions

Heat olive oil in a medium pan over a high flame

Add vegetables to the pan and turn sporadically; cook for 15 minutes

Add beans, tomatoes, and vinegar to vegetables and simmer for 5 minutes

Set couscous into a bowl and add vegetable stock

Stir for 3 minutes

Pour the couscous into a bowl and top off with the vegetable mixture

5.51   Polenta Arepas (vegan)

Ingredients

8 Ounces of Tofu

16 Ounces of Polenta

½ Tablespoon of Olive Oil

½ Banana

1/4 Cup of Black Beans

½ Avocado

1 Tablespoon of Onion

1/4 Mango

¼ Jalapeno

Salt and Pepper to taste

Directions

Preheat your oven's broiler

Slice up tofu and polenta and brush them with olive
oil before arranging them and a baking sheet

Cook them in the broiler for 5 minutes

Heat olive oil in a skillet and sauté bananas for 5 minutes

Place black beans into a blender and process them until they have become a sauce

In a bowl, combine onion, mango, salt and pepper, and jalapeno

Set polenta and tofu on a plate and cover them with the bean sauce

Add bananas and the mixture; top off with salsa and serve

5.52 CHICKPEA CASSEROLE

Ingredients

1 Teaspoon of Olive Oil

1 Can of Chickpeas

½ Cup of Water

¼ Cup of White Wine

2 Teaspoons of Chili Powder

1 Teaspoon of Red Pepper Flakes

2 Cups of Rice

Directions

Drain out the beans and place all of the ingredients
into a crock pot over a medium heat

Cook for 1 hour and serve

5.53 TEMPEH FAJITAS

Ingredients

1 ½ Teaspoon of Olive Oil

8 Ounces of Olive Oil

2 Teaspoons of Soy Sauce

1 Teaspoon of Lime Juice

1 Tablespoon of Onion

1 Clove of Garlic

1/3 Cup of Green Bell Pepper

¾ Teaspoon of Green Peppers

1 Tablespoon of Cilantro

2 Tortillas

Directions

Preheat your oven to 350 Degrees Fahrenheit

Heat oil in a skillet over a medium flame

Add garlic and onion; sauté for 3 minutes

Add soy sauce, lime juice, and tempeh and cook until browned

Add chile peppers, bell peppers, and cilantro and cook for 10 minutes

Heat corn tortillas in oven for 3 minutes

Fill up the tortillas with the mixture and serve

5.54 CHICKEN TERIYAKI STIR FRY

Ingredients

3 Ounces of Chicken Cubes

2 Teaspoons of Brown Sugar

1 Tablespoon of Honey

1 Cup of Rice

1/2 Cup of Bell Pepper Strips

1/3 Cup of Corn

Directions

Marinate the chicken cubes overnight in plastic bags in a marinade of brown sugar, sesame oil, and honey

Cook the next morning until complete and stir fry with corn, peppers, and rice; serve

5.55 KALE, LENTIL, AND RED ONION PASTA

Ingredients

½ Cup of Vegetable Broth

2 Tablespoons of Lentils

Salt and Pepper to taste

½ Leaf of Bay

1 Tablespoon of Olive Oil

¼ Red Onion

¼ Teaspoon of Chopped Thyme

1 Teaspoon of Dried Oregano

1 Vegan Sausage

¼ Bunch of Kale

1 Cup of Rotini Pasta

Directions

Boil bay leaves, vegetable brother, salt and pepper, and lentils in a sauce pan over a high flame

Reduce heat and cook for twenty minutes

Add vegetable broth and discard the bay leaves

Heat olive oil in a separate skillet over a medium flame

Stir in thyme, onion, oregano, salt and pepper

Add sausage and reduce heat; cook for 10 minutes

Boil a pot of salted water and add rotini pasta and kale

Cook for 8 minutes

Drain the pasta and add in the onion mixture and lentils and serve

5.56 BUTTER FETTUCINE

Ingredients

4 Ounces of Fettucine

½ Tablespoon of Melted Butter

1 Teaspoon of Basil

1 Teaspoon of Thyme

1 Teaspoon of Oregano

Directions

Cook the fettucine for 8 minutes

Mix the melted butter with thyme, oregano, and basil

Pour this mixture over the fettucine and serve

5.57 TERIYAKI TOFU AND PINEAPPLE

Ingredients

12 Ounces of Package Tofu

1/3 Cup of Pineapple

½ Cup of Teriyaki Sauce

¼ Cup of Rice

Water

Directions

Cut up the tofu and place in a dish

Add pineapple and teriyaki sauce

Cover and refrigerate for one hour

Preheat oven to 350 degrees Fahrenheit

Bake tofu for 20 minutes

Place rice and water in a pot and boil over a high

flame before reducing heating and simmering for 15

minutes

Pour rice into a bowl and top off with the pineapple teriyaki tofu and serve

5.58 TORTILLAS AND RICE

Ingredients

2 Cups of Cooked Rice

Olive Oil to taste

½ Tablespoon of Chili Powder

½ Teaspoons of Cumin

2 Tortilla Shells

Directions

Preheat oven to 400 degrees Fahrenheit

Place rice on a stove and add water and spices

Boil and then reduce the heat and simmer for 25 minutes while stirring

Set the tortilla shells over one another and cut into triangles

Set the tortilla pieces on the baking tray and cook for 22 minutes

Remove from tray, cover with the rest of the mixes, and serve

5.59 Tofu and Red Bell Peppers

Ingredients

14 Ounces of Tofu

½ Tablespoon of Olive Oil

½ Tablespoon of Soy Sauce

½ Red Bell Pepper

1 Tablespoon of Onion

¾ Tablespoon of Peanut Butter

½ Tablespoon of Lime Juice

2 Teaspoons of Sriracha

2 Teaspoons of Brown Sugar

Water

½ Tablespoons of Cilantro

Directions

Start by preheating your oven to 450 degrees Fahrenheit

Slice the tofu into four square like pieces

Whisk olive oil and soy sauce in a bowl

Coat the tofu in the resulting mixture

Place the pieces of tofu on a baking sheet and place onions and peppers alongside them

Bake for 10-15 minutes

In a pan over a low flame, mix together lime juice, peanut butter, chili sauce, brown sugar, soy sauce, and water; cook until warm

Remove the tofu, onions, and peppers from the oven and set in a bowl

Cover it with the new peanut butter mixture and top with cilantro if desired before serving

5.60 BROCCOLI CURRY

Ingredients

½ Tablespoon of Vegetable Oil

2/3 Cup of Broccoli

1 Cup of Rice

½ Cup of Water

1 Tablespoon of Coconut Milk

2 Tablespoons of Turmeric

Directions

Pour oil in a pot over a medium flame and sauté broccoli and tofu for 3 minutes

Add water, rice, coconut milk, and boil

Lower heat and simmer for 30 minutes

Stir in rice and serve

5.61 RISOTTO

Ingredients

3 Ounces of Ham (low sodium)

1 Tablespoon of Butter

1 Tablespoon of Olive Oil

2 Cups of Rice

1 Cup of Vegetable Bouillon

1/3 Teaspoon of Black Pepper

¼ Teaspoon of Orange Peel

2 Scallions

Directions

Melt butter and pour it into olive oil in a skillet over

a medium heat

Pour in uncooked rice and stir it for 5 minutes

Add the ham, spices, and bullion

Increase the heat and bring the mixture to a boil

Top off with scallions and serve

5.62 ALMOND AND QUINOA SALAD

Ingredients

3 Tablespoons of Almonds

¼ Cup of Quinoa

Water

2 Teaspoons of Olive Oil

½ Yellow Bell Pepper

1 Clove of Garlic

Salt and Pepper

Lime Juice

Directions

Preheat oven to 350 Degrees Fahrenheit

Set the almonds on a baking sheet and bake in the oven for seen minutes

In a pan over a medium flame, heat a teaspoon of olive oil

Add garlic, scallions, yellow pepper, and red pepper flakes and cook for five minutes

Add salt and pepper, water, thyme, and quinoa and boil before reducing heat of flame to simmer for 7 minutes

Add in zucchini and stir and cook for five more minutes

Remove the pan from the heat and add celery, almonds, and olive oil

Season with salt and pepper and continue to stir before serving

5.63 Tofu Fajitas

Ingredients

4 Tortilla Shells

½ Tablespoon of Butter

1 Tablespoon of Coconut Oil

1 Onion

2 Bell Peppers

1 Block of Tofu

2 Teaspoons of Lemon Juice

1 Teaspoon of Cayenne Pepper

½ Teaspoon of Cumin

Directions

Warm the shells in a skillet for 2 minutes

Cut the onions, tofu, and peppers into strips

Slather them with butter in a large pot and cook over a high heat for 3 minutes

Add this mixture over the shells and serve

5.64 VEGAN CHILI

Ingredients

2 Tablespoons of Olive Oil

1 Onion

4 Cloves of Garlic

1 ½ Teaspoon of Cumin

1 Teaspoon of Chili Powder

Salt and Pepper

1 Zucchini

¾ Cup of Tomato Paste

15 Ounces of Black Beans

15 Ounces of Pinto Beans

1 can of Tomatoes

Water

Directions

Heat the olive oil in a pot over a high flame

Add garlic and onion and cook for 4 minutes

Add chili powder, cumin, and salt and pepper

Add zucchini and tomato paste and cook for 3 minutes

Add black and pinto beans and tomatoes, and two cups of water

Boil the resulting mixture

Bring heat down and simmer the mixture for 20 minutes

Serve

5.65 VEGGIE BURGER WITH CUCUMBER SALAD

Ingredients

1 Ciabatta Roll

1 Veggie Burger

1 Teaspoon of Brown Sugar

1 Teaspoon of Thyme

1 Onion

1 Cucumber

4 Cherry Tomatoes

3 Cups of Olive Oil

1 Shallot

1 Tablespoon of White Wine Vinegar

½ Tablespoon of Basil

Directions

Cut the cucumbers into crescent shapes and then cut the cherry tomatoes in half

Slice the onions into strips

Place the onion strips, cucumbers, and cherry tomatoes into a bowl and mix it with basic, vinegar, and olive oil to form a salad

Cover up the salad and store it in a refrigerator

Mix brown sugar and thyme and sprinkle it over a veggie burger

Cook the burger until complete

Retrieve the salad from the refrigerator and serve it alongside the veggie burger

5.66 SESAME TOFU AND BROCCOLI

Ingredients

½ Block of Tofu

1 Tablespoon of Sesame Seeds

¼ Tablespoon of Sesame Oil

¾ Tablespoon of Soy Sauce

1 Cup of Broccoli

Salt and Pepper

Water

Directions

Slice the tofu into two pieces and then into two pieces each to make four pieces total

Spread out all of your sesame seeds out on a plate

Press all sides of the tofu pieces into the square

Heat sesame oil in a skillet over a medium flame

Cook the tofu for five minutes on each side in the skillet

Add in soy sauce and cook for one more minute

Remove the tofu from the skillet, and then add water, broccoli, and salt and paper into the skillet and cook for five minutes

Place the tofu and broccoli on an eating plate and serve

5.67 POT PIE MUFFIN

Ingredients

3 Ounces of White Chicken Meat

1 Cup of Cauliflower

½ Cup of Chicken Bouillon

1/3 Cup of Vegetable Mix

1 Teaspoon of Garlic

1/8 Teaspoon of Sage

Directions

Preheat oven to 375 degrees Fahrenheit

Place cauliflower in a food processor and process

In a bowl mix together mash, seasonings, and chicken

Set the dough on a flat surface and cut it up into holes that can fit in a muffin mold tray

Fill up each muffin with a spoonful of the mixture

Bake for 20 minutes and serve

Ingredients

1 Sweet Potato

¼ Tablespoon of Olive Oil

¼ Onion

1 Clove of Garlic

½ Teaspoon of Rosemary

1 Pinch of Red Pepper Flakes

Salt and Pepper to Taste

1 Cup of Kale

2 Ounces of Tofu

Water

Directions

Preheat your oven to 375 degrees Fahrenheit

Bake your sweet potato on a baking sheet for 1 hour, but keep the oven on

Cut off the top quarter of the potato and throw it away to leave a shell

Heat oil in a skillet over a high flame and add onion, rosemary, salt and pepper, garlic, and red pepper flakes

Cook while stirring for 3 minutes

Add kale and cook for 5 more minutes

Add in sweet potato, tofu, and water

Cook for 1 more minute

Place the entire meal on baking sheet and bake it for 30 minutes before serving

5.68 VEGGIE PITA

Ingredients

1 Pita Pocket

1 Teaspoon of Paprika

¼ Teaspoon of Black Pepper

1/3 Cup of Bok Choy Pieces

1/3 Cup of Avocado Pieces

1/3 Cup of Cucumber

1/3 Cup of Carrots

1/3 Cup of Tomatoes

1 Teaspoon of Lemon Juice

Directions

Begin heating your boiler

Place the vegetables into a bowl and add lemon juice and spices

Mix the vegetables and spices together well

Spoon this mix inside the pita and cook in the broiler for 5 minutes before serving

5.69 TOFU KEBABS AND CILANTRO

Ingredients

½ Cup of Cilantro

1 Tablespoon of Olive Oil

¼ Jalapeno

1 Teaspoon of Ginger

½ Tablespoon of Lime Juice

1 Scallion

Salt and Pepper

7 Ounces of Tofu

½ Squash

Directions:

Heat up your grill to medium heat

Combine oil, cilantro, jalapeno, ginger, juice, and scallion together in a processor

Blend until the mixture is smooth and then add salt and pepper

In a bowl, combine tofu, scallions, and olive oil

Place the scallions and tofu into a skewer and then the squash into another skewer

Grill the resulting squash kebab for 12 minutes over the grill and the tofu kebab for 7 minutes

Season with cilantro and serve

5.70 CHICKEN NUGGETS AND CHINESE VEGGIE SALAD

Ingredients

3 Ounces of Chicken Meat

2 Egg Whites

Salt and Pepper

2 Cups of Cabbage

Salt and Pepper

1 Stalk of Bok Choy

3 Ounces of bean Sprouts

Directions

Preheat Oven to 375 Degrees Fahrenheit

Scramble up your eggs in a bowl, and then your seasoning and breadcrumbs in another mixture

Run the chicken through the egg coating and the breadcrumb/seasoning coating

Set the chicken on a baking tray and cook for 25 minutes and then serve

5.71 VEGAN SALAD

Ingredients:

¼ Cup of Amaranth

1/2 Cup of Vegetable Broth

½ Cup of Quinoa

¼ Teaspoon of Orange Zest

¼ Cup of Orange Segments

¼ Cup of Fennel

¼ Cup of Radishes

1 Tablespoon of Olive Oil

2 Tablespoon of Orange Juice

½ Tablespoon of Red Wine Vinegar

Salt and Pepper

Directions

Cook the amaranth by placing it in a pan over a high flame and toasting for five minutes

In a separate pan, bring a half cup of vegetable broth to a broil

Transfer the amaranth to the vegetable broth pain and simmer for seven minutes after reducing the flame

Remove pan from heat

Cook quinoa by also placing it in a pan of boiled vegetable broth and add salt and pepper; simmer for 10 minutes under a reduced heat after boiling

Cook the millet by placing it in yet another pan over a medium to high flame and cooking for five minutes

Pour the millet into a bowl and mix it with cold water

Bring more vegetable brother to a boil in another pan

Add the millet and salt to the brother and simmer for 15 minutes

Merge all of the ingredients into one bowl and refrigerate for 1 hour before serving

5.72 Pizza (Gout Friendly Version)

Ingredients

2 Tablespoons of Olive Oil

1 Cup of Feta Cheese

4 Cups of Cherry Tomatoes

1 Cup of Radish

1 Cup of Avocado

1 Teaspoon of Red Pepper Flakes

1 Tablespoon of Basil Leaves

1 Teaspoon of Oregano

Pizza Dough (enough as needed)

Directions

Flatten out the pizza dough and cover it with olive
oil, seasoning and cheese

Add the rest of the ingredients and bake according
to the instructions on the dough package

5.73 BARLEY AND WINTER GREEN PESTO

Ingredients

½ Cup of Barley

Water

½ Bunch of Swiss Chard

½ Bunch of Mustard Greens

2 Tablespoons of Almonds

1 ½ Teaspoon of Vinegar

1 Clove of Garlic

1 ½ Tablespoon of Walnut Oil

Salt and Pepper

Directions

Set the barley and salt and pepper on a pan

Boil the pan over a high heat, and then reduce the heat and simmer for 30 minutes

Drain the pan and then fill up another pan with salted water and boil it as well

Add chard and mustard green to this pan and simmer for 1 minute

Drain the second pan

Mix greens, vinegar, almonds, and garlic in a food processor and process

Add walnut oil into the mix and continue to process for 2 more minutes

Mix all of the ingredients together and add pesto and barley and more salt and pepper as desired before serving

5.74 GARBANZO CAKE AND AVOCADO

Ingredients

¼ Cup of Bulgur Wheat

Water

¼ Cup of Parsley Leaves

14 Cup of Mint Leaves

¼ Cup of Cilantro Leaves

1 Clove of Garlic

1/4 Teaspoon of Coriander

½ Jalapeno Chili

½ Can of Garbanzo beans

¼ Cup of Olive Oil

¼ Avocado

½ Tablespoon of Lime Juice

Breadcrumbs

Directions

Bring a cup of water to a boil

Ad bulgur wheat and cook for 10 minutes, and then drain

Mix parsley, cilantro, mint, garlic, jalapeno peppers, and coriander together in a food processor and process

Add half of the garbanzo beans and pulse again

Transfer the bean mixture to a bowl and add chickpeas and process again.

Transfer to the same bowl

Add bulgur wheat to the bowl as well

Season the chickpea/bean/wheat mixture in the bowl with salt and pepper

Fold the mixture with a spatula

Cut the mix into patties with each patty being an inch wide

Combine flour and water together in a second bowl and mix it together until smooth

Dip each patty in the mixture to coat it thoroughly and then cover both sides with breadcrumbs

Transfer the patties to a plate and cook in a skillet over a medium flame for about 2-3 minutes on each side

Season again with salt and pepper and limejuice, and serve alongside mashed avocado and onions

5.75 VEGGIE BURGER QUESADILLA

Ingredients

2 burrito tortillas

3 ounces of veggie burger

¼ Cup of Mexican cheese

½ cup of scallions

1 teaspoons of chili

½ teaspoon of cumin

1 teaspoon of cilantro

1 tablespoon of Mexican seasoning

Directions

Set a skillet over a medium to high flame

Layer the ingredients between the two tortillas to make a quesadilla

Cook the quesadilla on both sides in the skillet, with at least four minutes per side

Remove and serve

5.76 VEGAN PAELLA

Ingredients:

Water

¼ Cup of Rice

¾ Teaspoons of Olive Oil

¼ Onion

1 Clove of Garlic

¼ Green Bell Pepper

¼ Red Bell Pepper

½ Tomato

¼ Cup of Vegetable Broth

1 Teaspoon of Paprika

½ Teaspoon of Turmeric

¼ Cup of Beas

¼ Cup of Artichoke Hearts

Salt and Pepper

Directions

Mix the water and rice together in a bowl and let it
sit for 20 minutes before draining

Heat the olive oil in a skillet over a medium flame
and stir it for five minutes with onion and garlic

Add red bell and green bell peppers and tomato

Cook and stir for 3 minutes

Add rice and vegetable brother into the mixture and
boil

Reduce heat and allow to simmer, with an addition
of paprika and turmeric, for 20 more minutes

Add salt and pepper, peas, and artichoke hearts into the rice mixture and stir for 1 minute

Merge all remaining ingredients and serve

5.77 CELERY ROOT SOUP

Ingredients

3 Tablespoons of Olive Oil

1 Cup of Celery Root

2 Potatoes

1 Apple

2 Cloves of Garlic

Salt and Pepper

Water

2 Cups of Vegetable Broth

Directions

Heat the olive oil in a pan with a lid over a medium flame

Add celery roots, potatoes, garlic, salt and pepper, and apple and cook for three minutes

Add water and broth and increase temperature to a boil

Reduce heat and simmer the vegetables for twenty minutes

Pour the soup into a blender and puree it

Once the soup has been blended, transfer it back to the pan and warm it over a low heat

Add more salt and pepper, and serve

5.78 SPICY QUINOA AND EDAMAME

Ingredients

Water

½ Cup of Quinoa

1 Teaspoon of Vegetable Bouillon

¾ Cup of Edamame

1 Teaspoon of Olive Oil

½ Sweet Onion

½ Bell Pepper

1 ½ Teaspoon of Ginger

2 Cloves of garlic

1 Tablespoon of Soy Sauce

2 Teaspoon of Cilantro

1 Teaspoon of Hot Sauce

Directions

Mix vegetable bouillon, quinoa, and water together in a pot over a medium flame

Add in edamame and simmer for 15 minutes

Heat up olive oil over a medium flame and add in peppers and onions and cook for 5 minutes

Add in garlic and ginger and cook for 2 minutes

Add in soy sauce, chili paste, and cilantro and continue to mix for 5 more minutes

Merge all ingredients and serve

5.79 ROAST BEEF WRAPS

Ingredients

1 Sandwich Wrap

3 Ounces of Roast Beef

1 Tablespoon of Onion Dip Powder

1 Roasted Pepper

1 Tomato

1 Tablespoon of Apple Cider Vinegar

1 Teaspoon of Lemon Juice

1 Red Pepper

Directions

Layout your sandwich wrap

Mix the onion dip powder, mushrooms, veggie slices, apple cider vinegar, lemon juice, and red pepper flakes in a bowl

Lay your roast beef on the wrap and then place the above mixture on top

Roll up the wrap and enjoy

5.80 BLACK EYED PEAS AND COLLARD GREENS AND TURNIPS

Ingredients

¼ Cup of Rice

Water

½ Cup of Peas

1 Teaspoon of Margarine (soy)

½ Turnip

1 Tomato

1 Teaspoon of Balsamic Vinaigrette Salad Dressing

¼ Bunch of Greens

Directions

Place the peas into a container and cover it with water and allow it to sit overnight

In the morning, prepare your rice by placing the rice and a small cup of water into a small pot

Boil the rice over a high flame, and then simmer it for 15 minutes

Cover up the peas that were soaked in water overnight with new water

Boil it over a high heat, and then simmer it over a medium flame for 40 minutes

Heat the soy margarine in a skillet and add greens and turnip and salt and pepper cook for 3 minutes

Combine the two mixtures and stir for 5 minutes

5.81 HONEYED CORN

Ingredients

4 Ears of Corn

3 Tablespoons of Honey

1 Tablespoon of Melted Butter

2/3 Tablespoon of Apple Cider Vinegar

1 Tablespoon of Turmeric

Directions

Mix the honey, vinegar, melted butter, and turmeric in a bowl

Coat each corn ear with the mixture

Wrap the corn ears and grill for twenty minutes over a medium heat

Serve

5.82 BLACK BEAN QUESADILLA (VEGAN VERSION)

Ingredients

¼ Cup of Black Beans

4 Tablespoons of Tomatoes

1 Clove of Garlic

½ Teaspoon of Cumin

1 Pinch of Chili Powder

1 Pinch of Cayenne Pepper

Salt and Pepper

2 Tortillas

1 Tablespoon of Cilantro

1 Teaspoon of Olive Oil

Directions

Blend the beans, tomatoes, and garlic in a processor and blend until smooth

Add chili powder, cayenne pepper, salt and pepper, and cumin and blend until smooth again

Transfer this mixture to a bowl and add a tablespoon of tomatoes and cilantro

Heat the olive oil in a skillet and then set the first tortilla over the oil

Spread your mixture over the tortilla, and then place another tortilla over it

Cook the tortilla for 5-10 minutes and flip at least twice

Serve

5.83 BAKED TOFU AND ROASTED PEPPER

Ingredients

½ Diced Shallot

¼ Container of Tofu

Water

1 Tablespoon of White Wine

1 Teaspoon of Red Pepper Slices

Directions

Preheat your oven to four hundred degrees Fahrenheit

Pour the water, peppers, tofu, and shallots into a pot and bake for twenty minutes before serving

5.84 RED BELL PEPPER (STUFFED)

Ingredients

¼ Cup of Brown Rice

Water

1 Red Bell Pepper

¼ Onion

1 Clove of Garlic

4 Ounces of Black Eyed Peas

1 Leaf of Swiss Chard

Salt and Pepper

Directions

Preheat your oven to 350 degrees Fahrenheit

Boil brown rice and water in a pan over a high heat

Reduce the heat and simmer for 15 minutes

Set red pepper on a baking sheet and bake for 15 minutes

Heat olive oil in a skillet and then add garlic and onion, and stir for 5 minutes

Add the peas and chard, and cook for 5 more minutes

Mix in the brown rice, season with salt and pepper, and stuff this mix into the red pepper

Serve

5.85 Baked Pepper Taquitos

Ingredients

6 Tortillas

1/3 Cup of Monterey Jack Cheese

1 Cup of Tomatoes

1 Jalapeno Pepper

1 Teaspoon of Chili Powder

1/3 Teaspoon of Cumin

½ Teaspoon of Celery Flakes

Olive Oil to Taste

Your Choice of Chicken or Pork

Directions

Either use leftover chicken or pork or cook new meat now

Shred apart your choice of meat and preheat your oven to 350 Degrees Fahrenheit

Lay tortillas on a baking tray and mix together the
protein, cheese, tomatoes, peppers, and spices

Pour this mixture over your tortillas and then add
the meat

Roll and bake for 30 Minutes

Serve

5.86 WHITE BEANS AND CHARD

Ingredients

¼ Bunch of Swiss Chard

1 Tablespoon of Olive Oil

¼ Onion

1 Clove of Garlic

Salt and pepper to taste

7 ounces of cannellini beans

½ Cup of Vegetable Broth

1 Tablespoon of parsley

1 teaspoon of white wine vinegar

Directions

Remove the stems from the chard leaves

Stack up the leaves and cut them into small pieces

Heat the olive oil in a pan over a medium flame until it shimmers

Add the chard stems, garlic, onion, and salt and pepper to taste

Cook and stir for 8 minutes

Then, add the chard leaves, beans, salt, and broth and stir for 5 more minutes

Remove from the oven and add in vinegar and parsley to taste before serving

5.87 BAKED CHICKEN WINGS

Ingredients

3 Ounces of Chicken Wings

1 Cup of Molasses

½ Cup of Ketchup

1 Tablespoon of Mustard

½ Tablespoon of Honey

2/3 Tablespoon of Hot Sauce

3 Teaspoons of Cayenne Powder

1 Jalapeno Pepper

Directions

Combine ketchup, molasses, honey, mustard, hot sauce, and spices together and boil over a high flame before reducing the flame and simmering for half an hour to create a sauce

Prepare your crock pot and then insert the chicken

Pour the sauce over the chicken

Bake for two hours before serving

5.88 MISO SOUP AND NAPA CABBAGE

Ingredients

1 Teaspoon of Olive Oil

¼ Onion

1 Teaspoon of Ginger

1 Clove of Garlic

1/ ½ Cups of Vegetable Broth

½ Tablespoon of Soy Sauce

6 Ounces of Noodles

¼ Cabbage

½ Carrot

¼ Cup of Hot Sauce

Directions

Bring a pot of salted water to boiling over a high flame

Add noodles to the water and cook according to the directions listed on the package

Drain out of the water

Heat the oil in a pan over a medium heat until it is shimmering, and then add ginger, garlic, carrot, and onion and cook for 5 minutes

Increase the heat and add soy sauce and broth and stir thoroughly

Add cabbage and stir and cook for 5 minutes

Add all of the ingredients together and season with salt and pepper as desired before serving

5.89 STUFFED PEPPER MELT

Ingredients

4 Bell Peppers

1 Tablespoon of Coconut Oil

1 Cup of Cauliflower

Scallions

1 Tablespoon of Mushrooms

1 Jalapeno Pepper

1 Cup of Monterey Jack Cheese

Directions

Preheat oven to 325 degrees Fahrenheit

Mix together all of the ingredients except for the cheese in a bowl

Spoon this mixture into the peppers

Top off with cheese and bake for 25 minutes before serving

5.90 CHINESE PORRIDGE (VEGAN VERSION)

Ingredients

Water

½ Cup of Vegetable Broth

½ Cup of Rice

¼ Piece of Ginger

Salt and Pepper

1 Cup of Kale

Directions

Place all of the ingredients except for the kale into a pan and boil it over a high flame

Reduce the flame and then simmer while stirring for one and a half hours

Shut off the heat and add the kale

Stir and cook for 5 minutes

Add more salt and pepper as desired and serve

5.91 ROASTED CHICKEN AND WHITE PEPPER

Ingredients

5 Pounds or Chicken

1/3 Cup of Olive Oil

½ Tablespoon of Sage

1 Teaspoon of White Pepper

1 Teaspoon of Rosemary

1 Teaspoon of Orange

Directions

Preheat oven to 350 degrees Fahrenheit

Place chicken in a dish

Mix oil, sage, oranges, peppers, and rosemary in a bowl and cook for one and a half hours before serving

5.92 SWISS CHARD AND GARBANZO BEANS

Ingredients:

2 Tablespoons of Nuts

4 Tablespoons of Couscous

1 Tablespoon of Olive Oil

1 Clove of Garlic

5 Tablespoons of Garbanzo Beans

2 Tablespoons of Raisins

¼ Bunch of Swiss Chard

Salt and Pepper

Directions

Set the couscous in a bowl and add water

Stir for 10 minutes

Cover this mixture and cook over a medium flame

While it is cooking, toast your nuts in a skillet over

a low heat for 3 minutes

Heat olive oil in a skillet and add garlic, garbanzo

beans, raisings, salt and pepper, and chard

Cook for 5 minutes

Fluff the couscous and place in a bowl; then top with previous mixture and nuts

5.93 GARBANZO CURRY

Ingredients:

¾ Teaspoon of Olive Oil

¼ Onion

½ Clove of Garlic

¼ Teaspoon of Ginger Root

1/8 Teaspoon of Cinnamon

1/8 Teaspoon of Cumin

1.8 Teaspoon of Coriander

1/8 Teaspoon of Cayenne Pepper

¼ Can of Garbanzo Beans

1/8 Teaspoon of Ground Turmeric

2 Tablespoons of Cilantro

¼ Cup of Rice

Water

Directions

Place water and rice in a pot and boil over a high heat

Reduce heat and simmer for 15 minutes

Heat olive oil in a skillet over a medium heat

Saute onions in olive oil for 3 minutes

Add garlic, ginger, cinnamon, cumin, salt and pepper, cayenne, coriander, and turmeric and cook for 1 minute while stirring

Add beans and water and cook for 15 minutes

Place rice in a bowl and top off with the mixture and cilantro

5.94 Peaches with Berry Sauce Ice Cream

Ingredients

Berry Sauce of your choice

Sliced Peaches

1 Tablespoon of Honey

1 Teaspoon of Lemon Juice

Low Fat Ice Cream of Your Choice

Directions

Scoop up ice cream in a bowl

Top off with all of the other ingredients and serve

5.95 Cornflake and Berries Cereal

Ingredients:

1 Cup of Frozen Berries

2 Cups of Cornflakes

1 Cup of Milk

Directions:

Pour milk into a bowl

Add cornflakes and berries and serve

6 CONCLUSION

Gout is a condition caused by a buildup of uric acid causing inflammation and irritation in your joints resulting in pain, swelling, stiffness, redness, and heat. With the help of some lab testing, your functional health doctor or other healthcare provider can help to determine your risk factors and underlying causes of gout and offer a personalized treatment plan to support your body naturally.

www.ingramcontent.com/pod-product-compliance
Lightning Source LLC
Chambersburg PA
CBHW061040250726
48653CB00001B/182